CU00937934

HOW TO CURE COLD SORES

UNRAVELLING THE COLD SORE MYTH

BY
JESSE ABBOTT

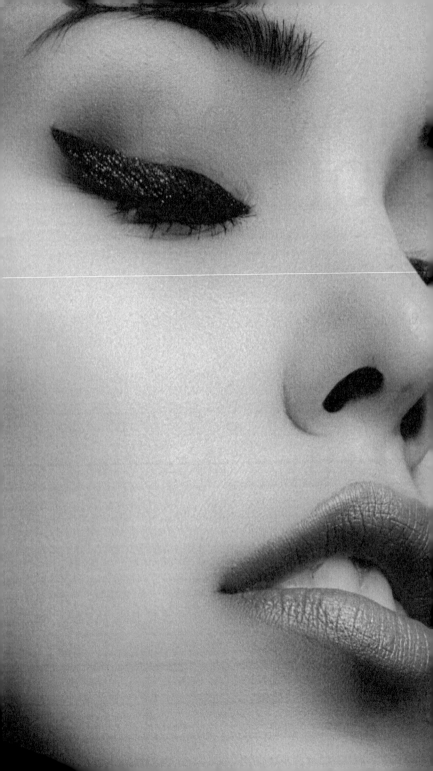

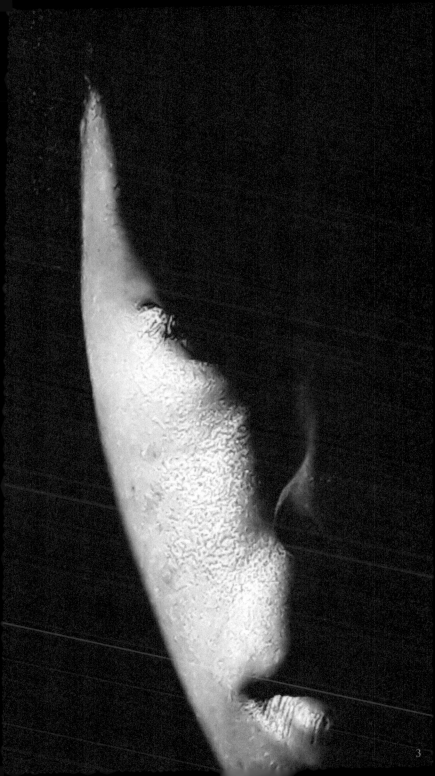

3

HOW TO CURE COLD SORES

Unravelling the cold sore myth

BY
JESSE ABBOTT

2024

CHAPTER 1
SHORT INTRO ON AWKWARD SITUATIONS

You would be surprised how easy it is to get a cold sore. And even more surprised how easy it is to NOT get one – EVER! Be protected for your entire life and present your best self, happy with ideal skin and glowing appearance.

Whether it's a job interview or an upcoming vacation, cold sores ALWAYS come at the worst times.

Most likely, at this point, you have had enough.

Enough of cold sores, enough of pimples, enough of skin imperfections, enough of not looking your absolute best. Enough of battling insecurities and worrying what nasty surprise your face, skin and body will surprise you with next.

You have picked up this book looking for answers and one place with the solution to all your anxieties in this area. You will learn how to treat your immediate cold sore concerns and be given a long term strategy to prevent any cold sore from appearing – EVER!

Then you will share this knowledge with your friends and family and become the beacon of health and pristine hygiene among your peers. This will allow you to demonstrate by example and know exactly what to do and what NOT to do to ENSURE YOU NEVER HAVE A COLD SORE AGAIN.

Imagine being able to live in a world free of cold sores? Now you have that opportunity, and this book will explain to you precisely and step-by step HOW to do it.

This book is intended for anyone that has ever had a cold sore, or knows someone that has. They cause anxiety, self doubt, pain, lasting damage, and are damn right ugly.

Let's get started with the cleanup.

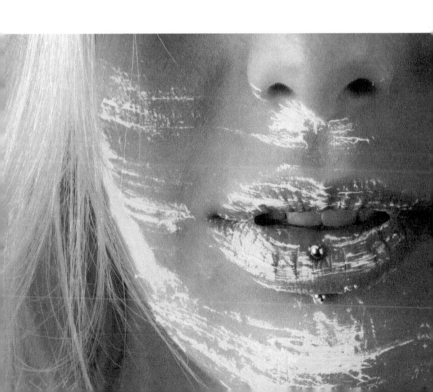

CHAPTER 2
COLD SORES

My name is Jesse, and I get cold sores.

Or at least I used to.

I have spent over 20 years trying to find ways to cure them, relieve th
pain, reduce how long they last, get rid of the embarrassment and be ab
to get on with my life.

I started just like you – annoyed, unaware and tried every solutio
under the sun. From coconut oil (which actually triggers cold sores!) t
prescription drugs to red light therapy to cold compresses to brande
goods sold in pharmacies – none of them work properly! More on these i
further chapters.

Over 70% of us have the virus that causes cold sores, but only aroun
half of us get those pesky cold sore outbreaks.

They can come at anytime, whether you've had them before or not.

They take anywhere from 1 week up to 3 weeks to clear up – and life i
no fun when you have them!

With the average cold sore sufferer getting 2 to 3 cold sore outbreak
per year, and each one lasting around 2 weeks, that's over 1 month out o
every single year that you have a cold sore!

We all get passed down strange folk tales on how to fix them, and in thi
book we will dispel those myths – and more importantly teach you hov
to never get cold sores again.

Thankfully, I have finally perfected the treatment of cold sore outbreaks, and more recently, even mastered the prevention of them altogether.

I am proud to say that I no longer get cold sores.

If you read the internet, it will tell you there is no cure for cold sores. This is not true. But to find that out, we first need to define that which we are fighting.

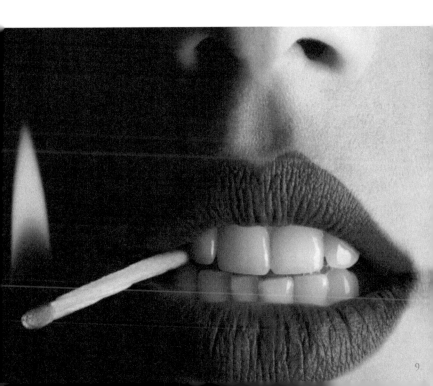

Chapter 3
WHAT IS A COLD SORE?

Cold sores, also known as fever blisters, are painful blisters that usually appear on the lips, mouth, and nose. They come out when the body has lowered immune system, and this acts as a double whammy because now the body has to fight them off when it is already struggling.

Cold sores are caused by the herpes simplex virus (HSV). Herpes Simplex Virus Type 1 (HSV-1) is a common and highly contagious virus that belongs to the herpesviridae family. It primarily causes oral herpes infections, resulting in cold sores or fever blisters around the mouth and on the face. HSV-1 spreads through direct contact with an infected person's saliva, skin, or mucous membranes. After the initial infection, the virus remains in the body in a dormant state, residing in nerve cells. Periodic reactivations can occur, leading to another outbreak of cold sores. HSV-1 is different from genital herpes (caused by HSV-2).

The scariest part is that once you have HSV, you will ALWAYS have it in your body, even if it may not always cause symptoms. It lays dormant most of the time, looking for opportunity and only causes cold sores when your body allows it too.

There is no way to remove this virus from your body, but what you can do is help your body fight any potential cold sore outbreaks. Your actions will prevent the virus from becoming the cold sores outbreaks that you hate.

Our bodies are complex systems of muscle, nerves, bones and host to a whole galaxy of bacteria and viruses, most are not harmful, but some are downright nasty, and those ones need to be kept at bay.

While your natural immune system maintains a pretty solid and stable alance, there are times when due to external influence or circumstances hat weaken it, you may contract illnesses, diseases and various ailments hat require intervention.

Ideally – you learn from this and maintain a lifestyle and habits that eep your health at an optimum state and use preventative methods to nsure your body is your temple of impenetrable fortress.

WHY DO WE GET THEM?
As with anything biological, multiple factors contribute to cold sores. Common triggers include:

Stress: Excessive emotional or physical stress can weaken the immune system, making it easier for the virus to reactivate and cause an outbreak.

Weakened Immune System: Illnesses, fatigue, or other conditions that compromise the immune system's function triggers cold sore outbreaks.

Ultraviolet (UV) Light Exposure: Overexposure to sunlight, especially on the lips, can trigger the reactivation of HSV-1 and lead to cold sores.

Hormonal Changes: Fluctuations in hormones, such as those occurring during menstruation or pregnancy, can trigger outbreaks in some individuals.

Trauma or Injury: Physical trauma to the lips, such as chapped lips, dental work, or injuries, can activate the virus and cause cold sores.

Certain Foods and Drinks: Foods high in arginine contribute to the growth of cold sores. More on this later.

How is HSV spread?

HSV is spread through contact with saliva or mucus that contains the virus. This can happen through direct contact with a cold sore, or through contact with objects that have the virus on them, such as a toothbrush or a glass.

Who is most at risk for cold sores?

People who are most at risk for cold sores are those who have had HSV infections in the past. People who are also at risk include those who have a weakened immune system, such as people that are run down or stressed. Children also tend to get them a little more often than adults.

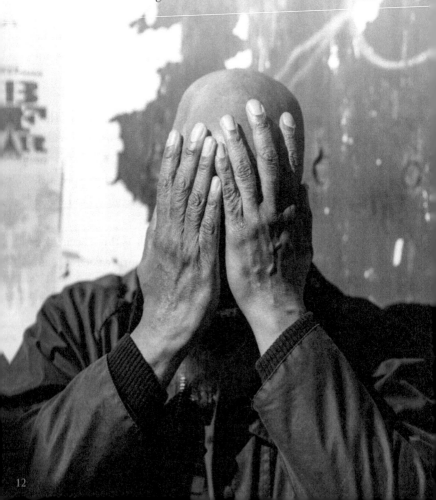

CHAPTER 4
FIRST SYMPTOMS

You know the feeling. The first tingle of pain, the awkward irritation n your skin that tells – you are now in for two weeks of embarrassment, discomfort and terrible inconveniences. You will never want to have this feeling again.

HOW IS DIAGNOSIS OF COLD SORES DONE?

Your doctor can usually diagnose a cold sore by looking at your blisters. They may also take a swab of the blister fluid to test for HSV.

However, most people that have cold sores regularly can easily tell as they are so very different from other outbreaks e.g. spots. If you get cold sores, you certainly know about it.

SYMPTOMS OF COLD SORES

The symptoms of cold sores may include:

1. Tingling (this usually comes first, and it is important to get used to this feelings so you can prevent the cold sore fully forming. More on that later.)
2. Redness
3. Burning
4. Itching
5. Pain
6. Swelling
7. Blisters
8. Inability of movement e.g. opening mouth/talking

They most commonly occur on the lips, but can also break out on the nose, inside the nose, inside the mouth, or anywhere on the face.

In rare circumstances they can also reach other parts of the body, causing major health issues including **encephalitis** (brain inflammation), **meningitis** (spinal cord membrane infection), **myopia** (poor vision), **neonatal herpes** (dangerous to newborns), **herpes simplex esophagitis** (inflammation in the throat) and even **blindness.**

Let's dive in to the dangers even more.

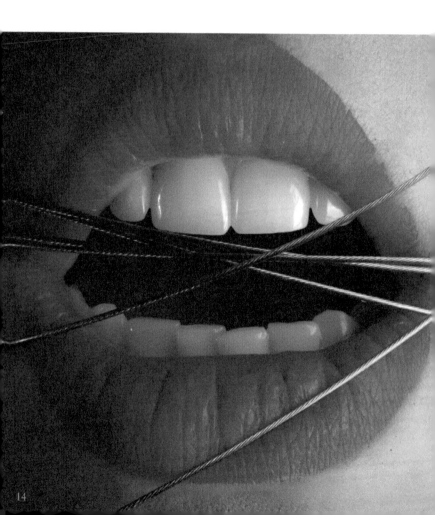

CHAPTER 5
WHAT ARE THE DANGERS
OF GETTING COLD SORES?

Cold sores can cause several potential complications, some of which re life threatening, and thus the need to avoid them altogether is even reater.

Cold sores can be painful and itchy, and people may scratch or pick at hem, which can cause the skin to break and become raw. When the skin s broken, bacteria can enter the sore and cause a secondary infection. Symptoms of a secondary bacterial infection may include increased pain, welling, redness, heat, and discharge from the sore.

The most common bacterial infection that can occur in cold sores is mpetigo, which is a highly contagious and unsightly skin infection. mpetigo can cause honey-coloured crusts to form over the cold sore, and t can spread to other parts of the body or to other people through direct nd indirect contact.

In addition to impetigo, cold sores can also become infected with other ypes of bacteria, such as cellulitis or folliculitis. Cellulitis is a skin nfection that affects the deeper layers of skin, while folliculitis is an nfection of the hair follicles. These types of infections can cause more erious symptoms, such as fever, chills, and even swollen lymph nodes ouch).

Cold sores are highly contagious, and direct contact with the sore can spread the virus to other parts of the body or to other people.

The virus can even spread through the saliva of an infected person, even if they don't have an active cold sore.

It's important to note that the herpes simplex virus can be transmitted even if there are no visible symptoms, as the virus can be shed from the skin or saliva without causing a cold sore.

It is very common (70% of spread cases), so you should be aware of it.

The virus can spread to other parts of the body or to other people through direct contact with the infected person or their personal items. For example, sharing a towel, razor, or utensils with an infected person can increase the risk of transmission.

The most common way that cold sores are spread is through kissing, which can allow the virus to be passed from one person's mouth to another. However, the virus can also be spread through oral sex, as the virus can infect the genital area and cause genital herpes.

If the cold sore spreads to the eyes, it can cause a condition called herpetic keratitis, which can lead to vision loss if not treated promptly.

Cold sores can be more severe, more problematic, and last longer in people with weakened immune systems. In these individuals, cold sores can lead to more severe symptoms and complications, such as widespread sores, longer healing times, and even life-threatening infections.

Cold sores can also be problematic for newborn babies, as they can cause a serious and potentially life-threatening infection (neonatal herpes). This can occur if a baby is exposed to the herpes simplex virus during birth, or shortly after, through close contact with an infected person.

Symptoms of neonatal herpes may include fever, lethargy, poor feeding, and skin rash or blisters. It is extremely dangerous.

There are also psychological effects. Cold sores are unsightly and cause mbarrassment or anxiety, particularly if they occur on the face or round the mouth.

Cold sores can have a significant psychological impact on people, particularly if they experience frequent or severe outbreaks. I for xample, used to avoid leaving the house altogether whenever I had a old sore. Sometimes I wouldn't even leave my bed! 10 days of not leaving he house? I'd rather avoid that altogether (and I now do).

The appearance of cold sores on visible areas such as the lips or face can e embarrassing and can cause individuals to feel self-conscious, anxious, r depressed. They may worry about being stigmatised or judged by thers, which can lead to social isolation and difficulties in forming elationships.

The discomfort and pain associated with cold sores can also interfere vith daily activities, such as eating, speaking, and smiling, which can mpact self-esteem and confidence. Most people avoid social situations r even work-related activities, which then makes the feelings of anxiety and depression even worse.

In addition to the immediate emotional effects, the psychological impact f cold sores can also have long-term effects. For example, individuals nay develop negative self-perceptions or beliefs about themselves, which an impact their overall quality of life and lead to depression or other nental health conditions.

WHEN TO SEE A DOCTOR
You should see a doctor if you have a cold sore that is severe, does not mprove with treatment, or is accompanied by other symptoms, such as fever, headache, or swollen lymph nodes.

However cold sores show themselves on your body, we can all agree li
is better without them.

Folk wisdom claims there is no cure for cold sores. Not true. There is r
cure for the HSV virus, which causes cold sores.

But the actual cold sores? You can stop them. You can make sure the
don't come out and never bother you again. I am living proof.

There is a way to prevent cold sores ever forming again. One more tim
as it's very important. **There is a way to prevent cold sores ever formin
again.**

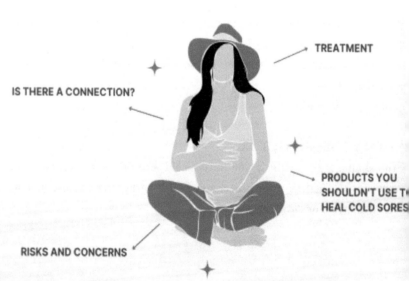

TREATMENT

IS THERE A CONNECTION?

PRODUCTS YOU
SHOULDN'T USE T
HEAL COLD SORES

RISKS AND CONCERNS

CHAPTER 6
RISK FACTORS FOR COLD SORES

There are a number of risk factors for cold sores, including:

Age

Family history

Weak immune system

Stress

Now let's go through each of these risk factors, and what you can do to reduce your risk of getting cold sores.

Age: well there's not much you can do about this, but cold sores are more common in younger people. This does not mean older people don't get them!

Family history: it is more likely you will have the cold sore virus if your close family members have it. 70% of the world has the virus, but not everyone shows symptoms (cold sores). If you're reading this book, I will assume that you or someone very close to you suffers from cold sores. The only thing you can do to prevent future generations getting the virus is to be very careful with them in their formative years and whenever they have open wounds when young. Most cold sores viruses are passed on from mother to child during childbirth, and there is not much we can do about that.

Weak immune system: Good news and bad news here. Your immune system is responsible for fighting off issues in your body. Most of the time the cold sore virus stays dormant, meaning it is there but not active. Your body is keeping it at bay. When certain triggers align, the virus will try to strike. One of these triggers is a low immune system. Ensure proper sleep, hydration, and enough vitamin C levels to keep your immune system strong.

- **Stress:** The silent killer. Stress affects everything negatively. There is tipping point, though. Stress can be what your muscles feel when yo lift a weight or go for a run. Your body's reaction to that stress is positive one. However, if you tried to lift a weight you could only li once, 1,000 times, it would not be good for you and your body wou suffer. A small amount of stress, and not having it constantly, can k good. Constant stress, or too much stress, is bad. When stress become severe (often referred to as chronic), it affects our body's ability t function properly in every way. Everything from your immune syster to your mental health is affected. How you view stress has a hug impact too, so try not to stress about the stress!

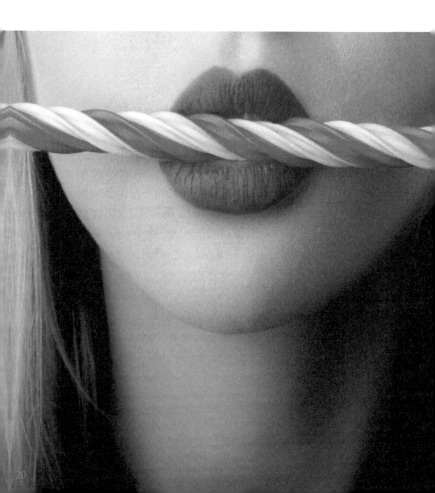

CHAPTER 7
TREATMENTS

Firstly, let's talk about treatments and how effective, or not, they are. Again, there's a lot of misinformation about this online. Most cold sore treatments are designed to reduce symptoms such as pain and swelling, and some do help, but there has never been a cure, up until recently.

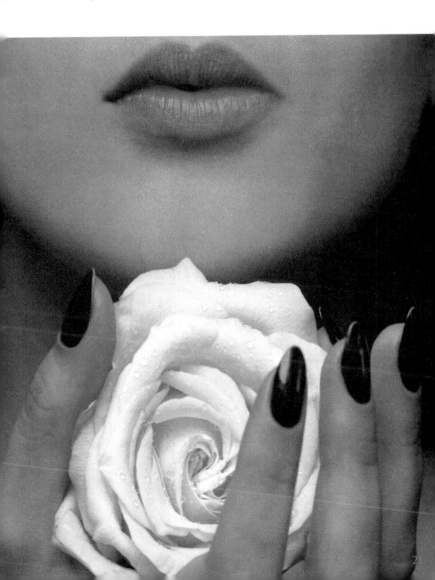

CHAPTER 7.1
MEDICINES

Common drugs such as ibuprofen and acetaminophen relieve pain and are sometimes used in cold sore outbreak treatment. They can obviously help with pain, but do not help with the cold sores themselves or the underlying causes.

Antiviral medications, designed to reduce the time the cold sore is present, include acyclovir and valacyclovir. These can reduce cold sore presence from 14 days to around 10 days.

There are a number of drugs that used to be used to treat cold sores. These include:

- **Acyclovir (Zovirax)** 60% approval rating
- **Valacyclovir (Valtrex)** 58% approval rating
- **Famciclovir (Famvir)** 72% approval rating
- **Docosanol (Abreva)** 45% approval rating

All ratings from drugs.com, correct at time of writing

These are all actual drugs and not natural treatments, so side effects can occur e.g. headaches. Another common thread amongst them all is they only have an effect when used before the cold sore has broken out.

So if you use a drug mentioned above to treat your cold sore before it breaks out, you may reduce the time you have a cold sore from 14 days to 10 days.

If you use the drugs mentioned above to treat your cold sore once it has already formed, you will see even less difference.

CHAPTER 7.2
NATURAL REMEDIES

There are a number of natural remedies that people claim can help to treat cold sores. But most do not have the desired effect. Let's start by dispelling the ones that are complete myths...

REMEDIES THAT DO NOT WORK

Coconut oil: coconut actually makes cold sores worse, due to its high arginine content!

Green tea: unfortunately this does not work. The hype was made by a company that used a disputed study, which used one molecule from within green tea, and claimed to reduce cold sore symptoms. The person that ran the study also owned the company. It doesn't actually work.

Cold compress: some call it applying a cold compress, some call it applying ice or an ice pack. Either way, the only potential benefit is reduced swelling, with no impact on the actual cold sore outbreak.

REMEDIES WITH POTENTIAL

Aloe vera: an important ingredient to soothe the skin, but by itself not enough to actually fight cold sores.

Lemon balm: another calming, soothing ingredient that can assist with symptoms of itching, burning and swelling, as well as virus spreading.

Tea tree: shown to help stop the cold sore virus, but can be harsh on the skin and dry out sensitive areas e.g. lips.

Zinc: Whilst not common, low levels of zinc can create issues for your immune system. Meat, seeds and fish are all good sources of zinc if you believe you have low zinc levels.

- **Vitamin C:** Very critical for a healthy immune system, the mo
important vitamin for immunity. Remember when a cold sore is tryir
to grow, it is a virus that is attacking your body and a healthy immur
system is necessary to fend off the attack quickly and successfull
(without symptoms ever showing). When you see a cold sore on yo
lip, your body has already lost the first few battles. The idea is to n
let it reach that stage.

- **Lysine:** Very important amino acid. If you have more lysine tha
arginine in your cells, cold sores cannot grow and replicate. Havin
more arginine than lysine is ESSENTIAL for cold sore growth an
replication. So, focus on the opposite, having more lysine than arginin

- **Calcium:** research has shown that having adequate calcium leve
prevents cold sores from forming.

- **Blackberry extract:** a study on blackberry extract showed that it ca
block early stages of HSV-1 growth and can directly kill the virus.

- **Astaxanthin:** when consumed, this directly exerts anti-oxidativ
activity to the skin that protects it from UV rays, which are a col
sore trigger.

Whilst these natural remedies helped me over the years, none wer
powerful enough alone to completely cure cold sores.

CHAPTER 8
PREVENTION

As well as the prevention, here are some things you can do to reduce your risk of infection.

PREVENTION OF COLD SORES

Everyone has a different circumstance, and so many different factors and lifestyle choices that all affect your body's immune system. All of this influences and can influence the way your body reacts to outside influences. While there is no immediate and 100% bulletproof way to prevent cold sores instantly, there are things you can do to reduce your risk of infection. These include:

Practicing good hygiene

Avoiding contact with people who have cold sores

Getting regular HSV testing

Good hygiene habits can help to reduce the risk of spreading HSV. These include:

Washing your hands often with soap and water

Avoid sharing personal items, such as towels and toothbrushes

Avoiding contact with people who have cold sores

If you know someone who has cold sores, avoid close contact with them when they are contagious. This means avoiding kissing, sharing utensils, and touching their blisters.

GETTING REGULAR HSV TESTING

If you are sexually active, it is important to get regular HSV testing. This will help you to identify any outbreaks early and to get treatment if necessary.

TAKING ANTIVIRAL MEDICATIONS

Antiviral medications can be a small help to reduce the risk of getting cold sores. These medications are available by prescription from your doctor.

WHEN TO BE EXTRA CAREFUL

When taking a flight or going on a long journey, when its extra sunny outside, when its extra windy outside, when you know your sleep will be affected – all great examples of when to be even more careful than usual. There is a cheat sheet coming up that will help you with this.

CONCLUSION

Cold sores are a common problem, but there are things you can do to reduce your risk of infection and to get treatment if you do get an outbreak. By following the advice in this book you can help to keep yourself healthy and cold sore free.

See the next chapter for a sure fire way to prevent cold sores appearing again.

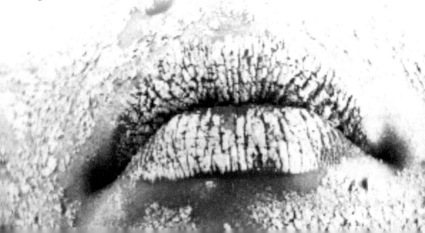

CHAPTER 9
PRODUCTS

There is a lot of research being done on cold sores. Some of the research is focused on finding new ways to prevent and treat cold sores. Other research is focused on understanding the causes of cold sores.

The research on cold sores is promising, but can be misleading. Research has helped us understand them more, but more research is always a good thing!

I used my expertise in the health research space mixed with years of painful trial and error to create the only 2 products you'll ever need to get rid of your cold sores forever.

We offer two products: **oldsore** and **helfi**. I recommend **helfi** and **oldsore** (two products from a company I own).

Ultimate answer in short: use **oldsore** oil to get rid of coldsores, use **helfi** supplement to prevent them coming in the first place and stay healthy overall.

Because I have tested them on me, I know they work. Plus thousands of others that use these products already. But I want this book to inform you, not sell to you. I want to cure cold sores for you, so it should be made clear that you do not have to buy **helfi** or **oldsore**. You can buy all the natural ingredients within them individually from any reputable, quality source.

Thankfully, there is now a 100% natural and healthy way to prevent cold sores completely. I developed an ingredient called "**helfi**" which contains L-lysine, vitamin C, blackberry extract, calcium lactate and astaxanthin. Each of these ingredients plays a role in ensuring a cold sore never forms again.

I went from 1 **coldsore** every single month, to zero cold sores ever wit
helfi. I take one sachet per day most of the time, and I double up to
sachets if I know I will be drinking alcohol or not getting much sleep.

I delayed the launch of this book until enough people were using hel
for a long enough period so that we could show you the results and rea
life experiences of people just like you and I, cold sore sufferers.

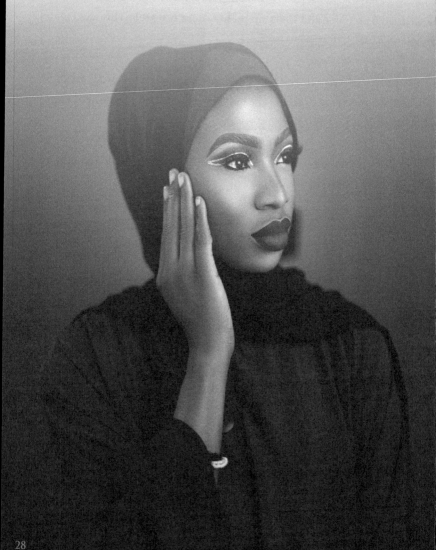

Chapter 10
Case Studies

IAM, UK, OLDSORE

Great product! This actually works! I can honestly say it has been a god
nd for me! I've had it for about 3 months and in that time I've had about
cold sores – every time I'm feeling a tingle I apply loads of old sore and
hen cold sore never becomes anything other than a small dry pimple. I
sually suffer bad with huge painful sores so this product has been life
hanging for me! Genuine review from a real human! Try it!

OAN, NEW ZEALAND, HELFI

I bought **helfi** as my son (13) started getting frequent coldsore outbreaks
oth inside and outside his mouth. He was crying a lot and didn't want
o attend school. Ever since he started taking 1 sachet per day, he has had
o coldsores, not even 1.

MELISSA, CANADA, HELFI

I am 57 years old, and am fortunate enough to have grandchildren that
love to spend time with. Whenever I had a cold sore I could not even go
ear them for fear of spreading it, let alone kiss them! I get more coldsores
n the winter usually, and average 4 per year. I tried using Abreva cream
nd aciclovir tablets, but nothing would make them better. My daughter
ecommended I try **helfi**, which I did. Since using helfi I have not had
ny coldsore outbreaks and can continue living my life without annoying
oldsores, meaning I get to see my grandchildren all the time. I now take
ny **helfi** everyday religiously!

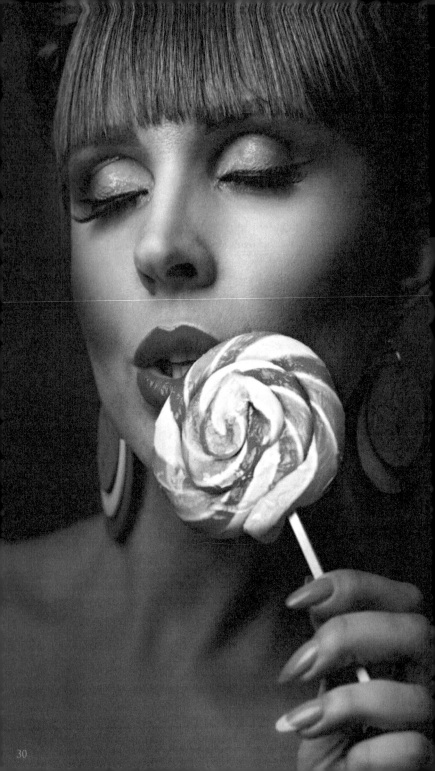

CHAPTER 11
HOW TO CURE COLD SORES

Now you can see the power of the daily **helfi** sachet, and this is the key to stopping cold sores ever forming again.

However, as powerful as **helfi** is, you want to be maximising your opportunity for health at all times. Not sleeping, being too stressed, flying a lot, drinking too much beer and wine... you are asking for trouble.

On the odd occasion that I now have problems with sleep and stress at the same time, I double up my **helfi** sachets (take 2 instead of 1) and keep a bottle of **oldsore** oil with me in case of a tingle.

Thankfully, my **oldsore** oils last longer than the best before dates as **helfi** does its job so well. At the time of writing I have not had a cold sore since starting to take the **helfi** supplement (over 2 years so far).

For reference I fly very often, and run multiple large businesses, so I am exposed to more sleep and stress issues than most. The supplement **helfi** has been a life changing one for me.

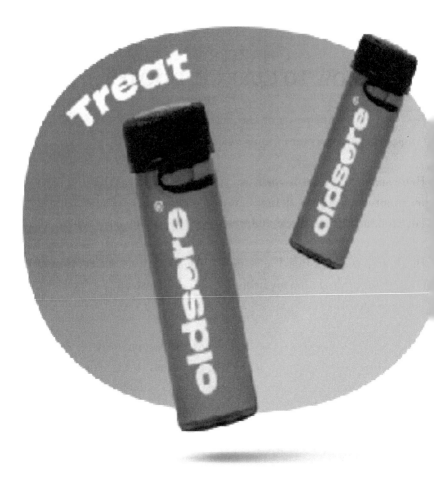

We have a product, called **oldsore**, it is a natural oil that is applied to a cold sore (preferably at tingle stage) to stop it forming. This is useful for those that don't like taking supplements and want to wait until a cold sore is forming before they deal with it.

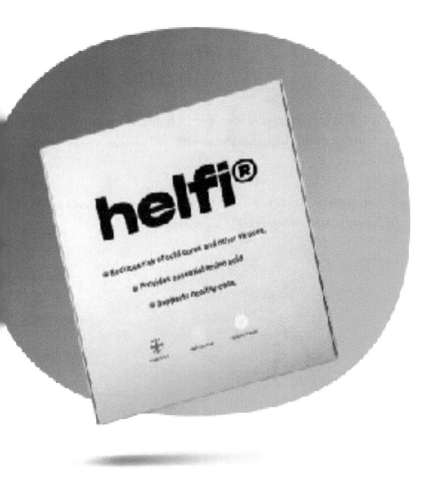

If you're like me and prefer to avoid cold sores altogether, **helfi** is the best option. I mix mine with a drink every day. It also has a number of other benefits including helping with bone health.

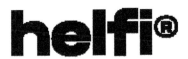

Chapter 11.1
Why helfi?

As well as preventing cold sores from forming, it has healthy ingredien
each with a double whammy (helps with cold sores as well as your gener
health).

Also, **oldsore** oil is fine to use on the lips, but some cold sores are INSID
the mouth, where **oldsore** oil is not recommended for.

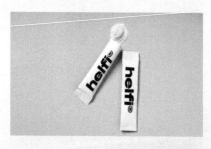

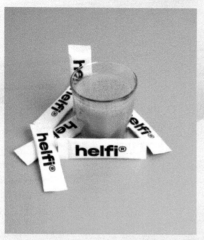

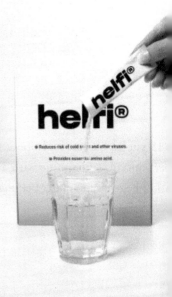

CHAPTER 11.2
OLDSORE

If you don't like taking a daily supplement, you can just keep a bottle f **oldsore** oil on you instead. This is to be used as soon as you feel a tingle, o stop the coldsore coming out.

The obvious and common advice is to keep good hygiene, such as hand ashing and avoiding people who have cold sores. These are wise, but ltimately most of us that get cold sores already have the virus and it just ares up at certain times. There are also medications claiming to be antiviral, ut they come with questionable effectiveness and some side effects. I tried hem all, and mostly I found them to deal with symptoms, not causes.

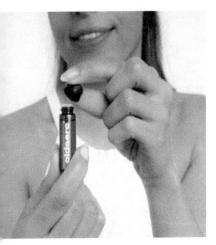
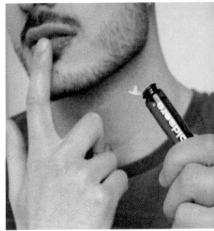
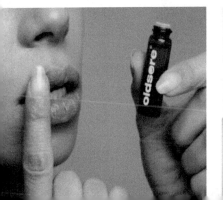
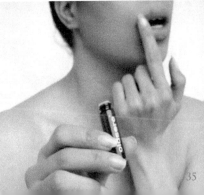

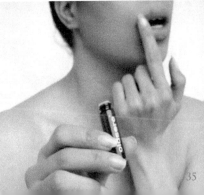

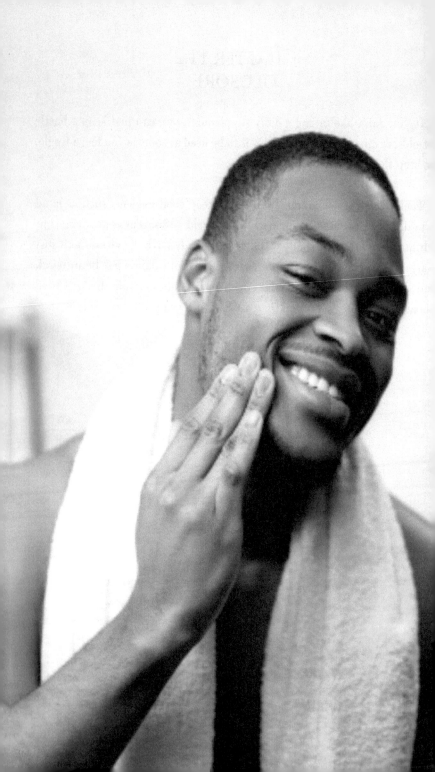

CHAPTER 12
WHO AM I

I have been taking **helfi** everyday since 2022 and never had a cold sore since. If I feel like I am starting to get run down, or I know I have a lot of flights or bad sleep coming up, I double the dose for a few days. **helfi** has never failed me.

I went from a dozen cold sore outbreaks per year, to zero. I am cured.

I am in a very fortunate position. I ran a health company for a number of years and it grew to be a global powerhouse. We did a lot of good in terms of research and science as well as making the best quality supplements (that actually work!) in the world. I did other things I consider good for the world, but they're not really relevant here. What is relevant is that I am already what I would call "rich", at least in monetary terms.

I was born on a council estate (a poor area) in England. So to now be a multi millionaire is beyond what I ever dreamed. I have invested wisely and made many, many millions. I am writing this very chapter on a private jet from the Galapagos Islands to Florida, USA. I feel a bit of a dick writing that, but it's true. I'm not sure if it's a British thing, but we find it difficult to talk openly about our successes for fear of coming across pompous and unlikeable. But I don't tell you this to brag, I tell you to make a point.

In short, I don't need your money.

I can also promise you that selling a product for £15 ($20) will not make you a lot of money. That's how much **oldsore** (the treatment) costs. **helfi** (the preventative) isn't much more. The running costs alone mean I would need to sell these products to a heck of a lot of people before turning a profit, and that's without the ever increasing postage costs and the cost of the highest quality ingredients.

I made **oldsore** and **helfi** because I wish I had had them all my life. Cold sores gave me great pain and anguish, and I want to solve problems in the world. If I am to be remembered at all, I want it to be for solving problems for humanity and the world. If you remember me only as the person that solved your cold sores, then I'll take that. If you don't remember me at all, but I helped to stop you ever getting a cold sore again, then I'm also happy with that.

I took a whole chapter to explain this because I think it's important. So, if you don't want to use **oldsore** and **helfi**, that's fine, just choose your sources wisely.

I mentioned my health research organisation. It gave me vast experience with supplements, and most of them do not contain what they claim to contain, so be very careful.

Amazon, for example, has literally zero quality controls. Every single supplement (over 50) that we bought from Amazon did not contain what it claimed on the label. P.S. we told Amazon several times and did not even get one single response. They do not care.

Please note: I expect other platforms to act exactly the same (e.g. eBay) so this isn't just an attack on Amazon, they are just the biggest player in the space at the time of writing.

So, if you are against buying from the person giving you the information, then get the ingredients for **helfi** individually (or maybe someone will have copied us by the time you read this) and use them. If money is no object, I recommend sending your product to a lab to get tested. If you can afford it then it is worth the peace of mind.

So in the next chapter, where I give you all the lifestyle alterations you eed to make to avoid cold sores ever again, when you see "take **helfi**" or use **oldsore**" – you can also think "or buy the ingredients individually rom a trusted source".

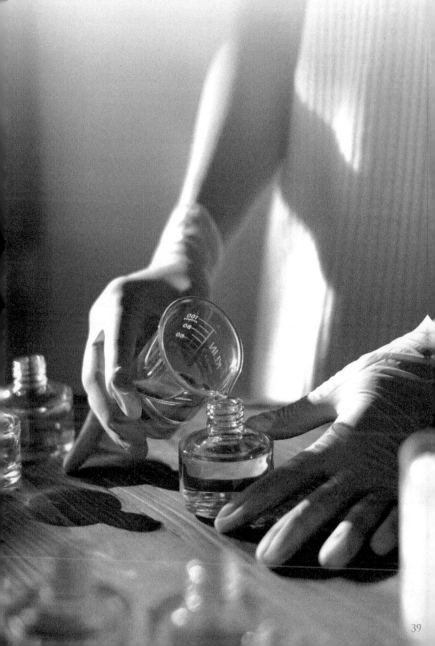

CHAPTER 13
INGREDIENTS

For your ease, the ingredients in **helfi** are written below:

- L-lysine
- Astaxanthin
- Blackberry extract
- Calcium lactate
- Vitamin C

And if you are not the type of person who likes to take supplements and prefer to let cold sores begin to form before you deal with them, the **oldsore** oil ingredients are below:

- Tea tree
- Aloe vera
- Peppermint
- Lemon balm

You may notice that these ingredients are a blend of the natural ingredients that showed promise in an earlier chapter. Perfecting the blends took a lot of trial and error, but eventually I found the perfect recipe to cure cold sores.

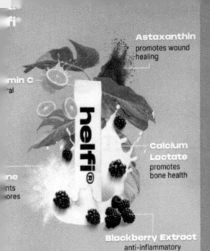

Astaxanthin promotes wound healing

Calcium Lactate promotes bone health

Blackberry Extract anti-inflammatory

---

olds●re

Blackberry Extract

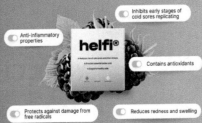

- Inhibits early stages of cold sores replicating
- Anti-inflammatory properties
- Contains antioxidants
- Protects against damage from free radicals
- Reduces redness and swelling

Did you know? Foods that are high in arginine, such as chocolate and nuts, should be avoided if you are prone to cold sores.

---

olds●re

Calcium Lactate

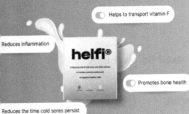

- Helps to transport vitamin F
- Reduces inflammation
- Promotes bone health
- Reduces the time cold sores persist
- Stimulates growth of new skin cells
- Speeds up healing process

---

olds●re

Vitamin C

- Reduces duration and severity of the outbreak
- Promotes production of white blood cells and antibodies
- Supports the immune system
- Protects the body's cells from free radicals
- Contains antioxidants
- Promotes healing

Did you know? Foods that are high in arginine, such as chocolate and nuts, should be avoided if you are prone to cold sores

---

olds●re

Lysine

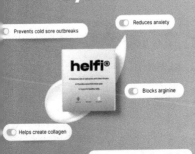

- Prevents cold sore outbreaks
- Reduces anxiety
- Blocks arginine
- Helps create collagen
- Prevents cold sores from replicating

---

olds●re

Astaxanthin

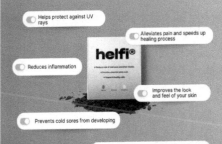

- Helps protect against UV rays
- Alleviates pain and speeds up healing process
- Reduces inflammation
- Improves the look and feel of your skin
- Prevents cold sores from developing
- Boosts the immune system by having immunomodulatory effects

YOUR CHEAT SHEET

Avoid food or drink high in arginine

- Nuts
- Bread
- Chocolate
- Beer

Avoid these too

- Stress
- Alcohol
- Poor sleep
- Too much sun and/or wind on your lips

What you should consume

- Avocado
- Cheese
- Meats
- Fish
- Beetroot
- Water
- belfi (supplement)

CHAPTER 14
CONCLUSION + YOUR CHEAT SHEET

This chapter is also known as the cheat sheet. Take a photo of it on your phone for ease.

Avoid food or drink high in arginine
  Nuts
  Bread
  Chocolate
  Beer

Avoid these too
  Stress
  Alcohol
  Poor sleep
  Too much sun and/or wind on your lips

What you should consume
  Avocado
  Cheese
  Meats
  Fish
  Beetroot
  Water
  helfi (supplement)

I have been taking **helfi** everyday since 2022 and never had a cold sore since. If I feel like I am starting to get run down, or I know I have a lot of flights or bad sleep coming up, I double the dose for a few days. **helfi** has never failed me.

I went from 10 cold sore outbreaks per year, to zero. Cured.

CHAPTER 15
HOW TO DO THIS IN REAL LIFE

Sometimes life gets in the way, and you cannot follow the above perfectly. For example if you are going to a celebration for the weekend. You will be drinking more than usual, and sleeping less. Or another example might be you feel you are getting sick. In these cases, do what you can to try and keep yourself safe from cold sores:

- Keep a bottle of **oldsore** oil on hand in case you feel a tingle

- Try to drink less alcohol, or at the very least choose spirits over beer

- Try to get as much sleep and rest as you can

- Reduce your stress, worrying about cold sores makes cold sores worse

- Stay hydrated

- Double your dose of **helfi** each day (take 2 sachets instead of 1)

- Give your lips extra protection from the elements by covering them or staying inside

You can get both the **oldsore** oil and the **helfi** sachets from www.**oldsore**.com – they are available anywhere in the world.

Stick with cheat sheet on previous page (print it out, write it down, do whatever you need to) and you will never get cold sores again.

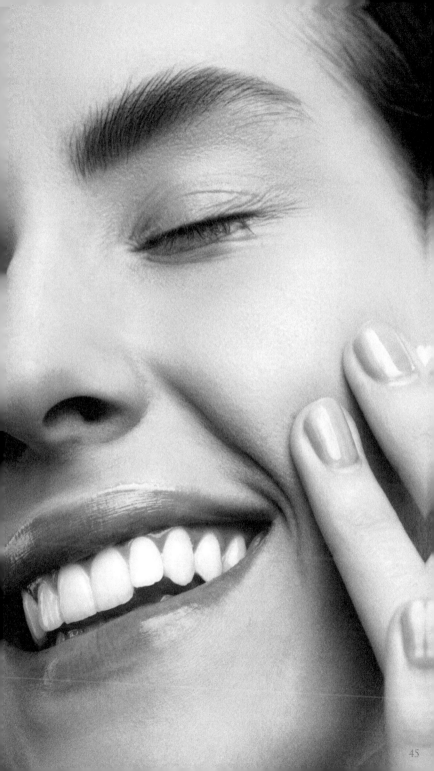

Note from the author

If you found value in this book, please consider leaving a review a▉ telling your friends and family about it. If you know someone that suffe▉ from them, consider buying a copy of this book for them as a gift, the▉ will be more thankful to you than you could ever imagine.

I hope the learnings that I have shared here have as positive an effe▉ on your life as they did mine. I am proud to say that I no longer get co▉ sores, and my mission is to ensure everybody else in the world can say t▉ same thing. In order to do that, this information needs to be shared.

We cannot cure viruses, but we can cure cold sores.

JESSE ABBOT▉

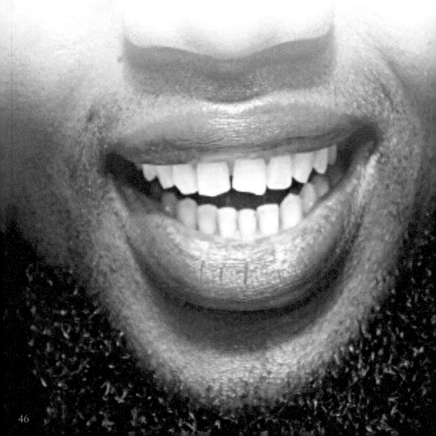

Appendix 1: Links

https://linktr.ee/**oldsore**   All links in one place

https://oldsore.com/pages/**helfi**   Shop **helfi**

https://oldsore.com/products/**oldsore**   Shop **oldsore**

https://www.**oldsore**.com   Website

https://**oldsore**.com/pages/contact   Contact

https://**oldsore**.com/products/**oldsore**?variant=43676515860798 Reviews

https://**oldsore**.com/#faqs   FAQs

https://instagram.com/_**oldsore**   Instagram

https://www.facebook.com/**oldsore**   Facebook

https://tiktok.com/@_**oldsore**   TikTok

Appendix 2: Reviews

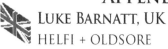
Luke Barnatt, UK
HELFI + OLDSORE

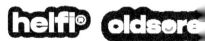

helfi, the ultimate savior of my confidence and success! It actually saved me money!

As a dynamic public speaker, content creator, and organizer of exclusive events for high net worth individuals, my professional life demands nothing short of perfection. But let's face it, those pesky cold sores have a knack for striking at the most inconvenient moments!

Countless times, these unwelcome intruders have threatened to sabotage my speaking engagements or even force me to miss out on important events. However, since discovering **helfi**, my life has taken a remarkable turn for the better!

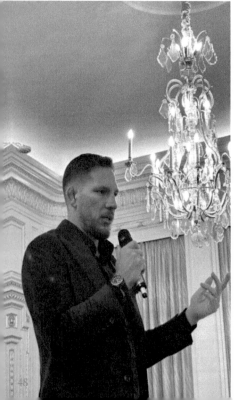

Just last week, after a grueling trip to Dubai where exhaustion had taken its toll, I woke up with that all-too-familiar tingling sensation. I knew that dreaded cold sore was about to rear its ugly head, and time was of the essence. Thankfully, I had my trusty **helfi** by my side (I never leave home without it now).

Without hesitation, I started my day with a powerful double dose of **helfi** sachets. But I didn't stop there. I religiously applied the miraculous **oldsore** treatment to my lip every 40-60 minutes as well, ensuring maximum protection.

And guess what? Another cold sore nightmare averted! With my worries put to rest, I soared to London for my event and delivered my talk with absolute peace of mind.

helfi has become my ultimate secret weapon in the battle against cold sores. Gone are the days of relying solely on L-Lysine, which I experimented with for years to no avail. **helfi** is the game-changer, the unparalleled solution that keeps me in control of my life and career.

I can't even fathom where I would be without **helfi**. It has become an indispensable part of my routine, empowering me to conquer cold sores and seize every opportunity that comes my way. **helfi**, you have my eternal gratitude!

SALMA YOUNIS, UK
HELFI + OLDSORE

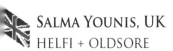 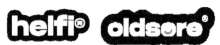

Having had cold sores for the forth time this year (previous years I got a cold sore once/twice a year). I have felt so desperate to treat and prevent any more cold sores coming. I came across **oldsore**. Was sceptical, but willing to try it – and it worked!!! As soon as I got a tingling, I applied **oldsore** nearly every hour – and within 2 days the cold sore was gone! It didn't even form properly or get to the scabbing stage. It has been amazing!

I hope I didn't just "get lucky" and it works every time, but I am hopeful it will. So far, if caught early enough, **oldsore** has worked quicker and more effectively than anything I've used so far... including Zovirax. Can't comment on how it will perform if the cold sore is caught after it has formed, which usually happens during the night.

Recommend this product!

HANNAH KING, UK
HELFI + OLDSORE

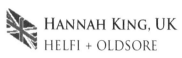 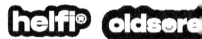

I've been taking **helfi** for a few months now and it's magic. I used to take lyseine and use all the topical treatments and would get a huge cold sore every 4-6 weeks, and one would try to come through every other week (I used topical and heat treatments to fight them back). I couldn't have chocolate, sugar, coffee or late nights as they would all bring them on!

Since using **helfi**, I've had NO coldsores! And when, in the early days, I had a couple try to come through, I used **oldsore** and they went away before they got to blister. I'm now enjoying chocolate, coffee and late nights, and zero horrid, itchy, embarrassing, painful, miserable coldsores. which is to say **helfi** has changed my life in a very positive way. Thank you

LINDA KRUPINSKI, UK
HELFI + OLDSORE

 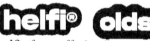

I've started my months supply of **helfi** after suffering 3 nasty cold sores last month, I took my first sachet as I was recovering from my 10 day cold sore, my lip feels and looks so much better, I feel confident that **helfi** will prevent further outbreaks.

PATRICIA TRIPP, UK
OLDSORE

 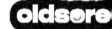

Cold sore was already established before this arrived. I used it every 45 mins (even set alarm on my phone). It did take a week to go, but usually it takes 3 weeks. It started drying up from the first application. Will never be without it and will hopefully catch the next one before it breaks out. Amazing stuff!

GEMMA HEDGES, UK
OLDSORE

 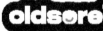

Cold sore was already underway, this arrived and applied it straight away and set my alarm to go off every 45mins! Dried it out so much quicker than other brands do. Will keep it in my pocket always!

LIA JAYNE GODDING, UK
HELFI + OLDSORE

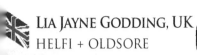 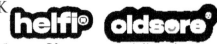

I have had cold sores for around 15 years, I have seen specialists, doctors and more... I really suffer when it's that time of the month or if Ive been out in the sun. I wear SPF50 on my lips! I'm even on Aciclovir tablets. I came across **oldsore** on a new hope and research of products and have been on **helfi** for a month and the ointment and I've had 2 coldsores try to break out and it literally has kept them at bay and stopped huge breakouts. I'm keeping my fingers crossed this keeps working, because so far it's been a life saver! Thank you, **oldsore**, from a very happy customer!

JOY CAVANAGH, UK
OLDSORE

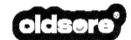

Totally sceptical, but thought: why not, give it a go…..

Yip, it works! When I arrive in the sun, I typically get a cold sore and have to nurse it along for a full week!!! Sure enough, arrived in holiday and there goes the tingle. I applied it immediately, and as often as I could remember…. It came up in a weird blister after 24 hours, but I kept applying and was amazed – the next day it was pain free. 48 hours to get the sting out… Maybe another 24-48 for it to disappear fully. Definitely recommend!

HANNAH BLAKER, UK
OLDSORE

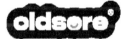

Life changing! I've suffered with coldsores for 40 years. When my bestie gave me a bottle of **oldsore** for my birthday, I didn't believe it would work... From the first application after the tingle I could actually feel the difference. It stopped the coldsore in its tracks.

I am beyond happy that I now have a defense against coldsores. One year I was in so much pain, I couldn't eat my Christmas dinner... no more ruined Christmas's! Thank you!

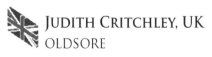 **JUDITH CRITCHLEY, UK**
OLDSORE

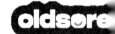

Don't dither, order now! I thought this sounded really good and was thinking about ordering it but dithered. Needless to say, the tingle started the next day! My order was delivered within 24 hours, too late to stop the coldsore... but it was certainly very good at speeding up the healing and stopping the pain.

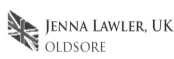 **JENNA LAWLER, UK**
OLDSORE

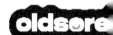

Fab product! Super effective! Highly recommend!

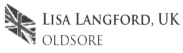 **LISA LANGFORD, UK**
OLDSORE

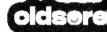

It actually works! I have suffered with cold sores all my life and have tried every treatment available. Recently, I have had one outbreak after another. Normally, it takes at least two weeks before they fully heal, sometimes longer. I tried **oldsore**, but was sceptical. The recent outbreak took three days to look so much better – and less than a week to be hardly noticeable. I will be buying more, and taking it with me everywhere

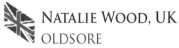 **NATALIE WOOD, UK**
OLDSORE

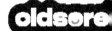

Saved my life! The day after my son was born in June, 3 coldsores appeared along my bottom lip! I then had them constantly for the next weeks! Being unable to kiss my new baby depressed me so much! **oldsore** saved me from the brink of crazy – all my coldsores were gone within days of using the product! I've not had one since, thank you so much!!!

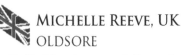 **MICHELLE REEVE, UK**
OLDSORE

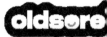

Baffled but impressed. I genuinely thought this was going to be a waste of money, but – with a giant face cold sore appearing about a week before

was due to meet new work colleagues for the first time – I thought was worth a shot. My cold sore was fairly developed by the time I'd ordered and it arrived... but I started putting it on the blister and it dried out so quickly. Somehow more impressive was: by the time it reached scab, when the scab came off, the skin underneath was fresh and pink – none of that multiple repeated scab nonsense that usually happens. Unfortunately, my cold sore spread and it got a new friend next door – I don't think the oil was to blame, more a run down immune system and trying to moisturise the remnants to speed up healing (a mistake!) – this oil sorted it right out in a few days. Not the 24hr fix it claims, but who knows – if you get it at tingle stage, then maybe. My bf, who gets cold sores regularly, was so sceptical, but is very impressed and is going to try it next time he gets one. 100% worth a try to speed up the healing process if nothing else!

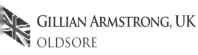 ### GILLIAN ARMSTRONG, UK
OLDSORE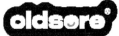

Sceptical, but impressed. Bought this after seeing ad on Facebook. I've had cold sores for years and few rounds of tablets from docs... the cold sores were so regular, I ordered this after the tingle so it was a bit scabby when started and they usually bleed/scab – this cleared it up in a few days, so much better than the usual 2 weeks plus. If you're not sure, definitely worth a try! It also arrived very quickly.

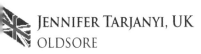 ### JENNIFER TARJANYI, UK
OLDSORE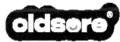

Sped things up. I have only occasionally suffered cold sores, then suddenly out of nowhere my whole top lip was covered! I'll spare you the photo, but it was full-on! I bought **oldsore** after the attack has started and was probably at its peak, but I'm convinced it dried them up and got them through scab phase quicker. And quicker than creams I've used in the past! They aren't going to just disappear overnight, but they quickly scabbed and came off with very little bleeding, at which point I switched

to a liquorice root lip balm from another supplier to help the dry sk
heal. Highly recommend, and will use at the first sign in future. I wor
waste my money on a pharmaceutical treatment again.

 ## JO STONES, AUSTRALIA
OLDSORE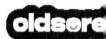

Definitely worth a buy. I've been getting 5 plus coldsores at once sin
being here in UK from Australia – this product definitely lessens th
length of the coldsore cycle – and dries them so well, gotta be relentle
with applying to get the full effect, and it's worth it. Recovery time is s
much better.

 ## MAIRI YOUNGER, UK
HELFI

It helped so much. Having suffered from these since childhood, wa
skeptical, but it stopped it in a few days, and the recovery was muc
quicker, thank you!

 ## GEORGIE GROCOTT, UK
OLDSORE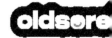

I'm impressed. So, I have started breaking out in a coldsore, 1 starte
putting this on as soon as I noticed the tingle and slight raised bum
(about a day and a half ago), I have been putting it on religiously ever
hour/2 hours while awake. My cold sore has already started healing to th
point it can't be seen, it didn't get to the puss/scab stage and I can say,
am really impressed with this stuff. I don't know what's in it, or how i
works – but I can tell: it's working for me! It really dries your lips, but I'r
trying not to put balm on, in case it spreads the sore. And I'm makin
sure to cover all my lip and skin just under it. It's not the 24 hour quic
fix, but I feel it is definitely working faster than the other supermarke
brands out there – and with a Christmas party coming up in a few days
I will keep applying to make sure it's definitely gone before the photos
I tried to take an image of the sore I have, but its so minimal you can'

ven see it on a close up anymore. I thought it would be a scam, this stuff
for it to be too good to be true, as the rest of this stuff is advertised.
Ionestly, I am converted and will be recommending it to others!

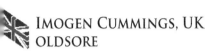 ## IMOGEN CUMMINGS, UK
OLDSORE

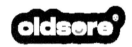

Absolutely amazing!

I never leave a review for any purchases I make but I had to make an
xception for this little bottle of gold! I was sceptical when I bought this
s I didn't think anything could cure a cold sore before it broke out. But
ow wrong was I.

I woke with the usual swelling on my lip & tingling yesterday & thought
h great just in time for Xmas (a week away) Applied this ointment
hroughout the day & it has disappeared the day after! This stuff is
imazing! 100% would recommend to a regular cold sore sufferer like
nyself! Wish I had found it sooner!

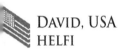 ## DAVID, USA
HELFI

My life became depressing after my cold sores took a turn for the worse.
When I get them they give me so much pain when I try and speak and eat
and drink. In the first half of 2023 I had 5 cold sore outbreaks.

I felt like I spent more time with cold sores than without. This is when I
started to use **helfi**. The coldsore I had disappeared straight away (I used
3 sachets on the first day), and I have not had a single outbreak since.

I have excelled at work since not getting cold sores and have a new
confidence. I feel a lot better in myself, I'm not sure if that is just the
lack of cold sores or the other benefits you get from **helfi**. Either way, I
am very grateful. Thank you.

Photograph References

Photo by Rodolfo Clix: https://www.pexels.com/photo/white-granule-on-person-lips-925802/

Photo by Rodolfo Clix: https://www.pexels.com/photo/woman-biting-gray-nails-in-her-mouth-1161930/

Photo by Rodolfo Clix: https://www.pexels.com/photo/woman-with-yellow-paint-on-the-face-1616002/

Photo by Rodolfo Clix: https://www.pexels.com/photo/woman-with-lighted-match-graphic-wallpaper-922511/

Photo by Rodolfo Clix: https://www.pexels.com/photo/closeup-photo-of-a-woman-with-gray-cables-on-his-mouth-1161935/

Photo by Rodolfo Clix: https://www.pexels.com/photo/woman-with-white-and-red-candy-cane-on-her-mouth-4416273/

Photo by Rodolfo Clix: https://www.pexels.com/photo/woman-holding-pink-rose-flower-1615841/

Photo by Oleksandr P: https://www.pexels.com/photo/close-up-photo-of-woman-holding-lollipop-1540408/

Photo by Alexander Krivitskiy: https://www.pexels.com/photo/gray-cale-photography-of-a-woman-s-face-1264442/

Photo by Raphael Brasileiro: https://www.pexels.com/photo/man-s-face-2401442/

Photo by Nicola Barts : https://www.pexels.com/photo/black-man-covering-face-with-hands-7926617/

Photo by Ricardo Garcia: https://www.pexels.com/photo/person-s-face-covered-with-white-powder-682501/

Photo by King Shooter: https://www.pexels.com/photo/a-woman-wearing-a-headscarf-19633033/

Photo by Anna Shvets: https://www.pexels.com/photo/crop-black-woman-making-aromatic-liquid-incense-5760907/

Photo by cottonbro studio: https://www.pexels.com/photo/person-holding-white-and-black-frame-4065183/

Photo by Shiny Diamond: https://www.pexels.com/photo/close-up-photo-of-woman-with-pink-lipstick-smiling-with-her-eyes-closed-3762408/

Photo by Keegan Checks: https://www.pexels.com/photo/smiling-man-in-black-jacket-and-wearing-sunglasses-4489863/